DEMENTIA

PRODUCTS USED AND EIGHT-PLUS YEARS CAREGIVING

Part of the Proceeds go to Charity

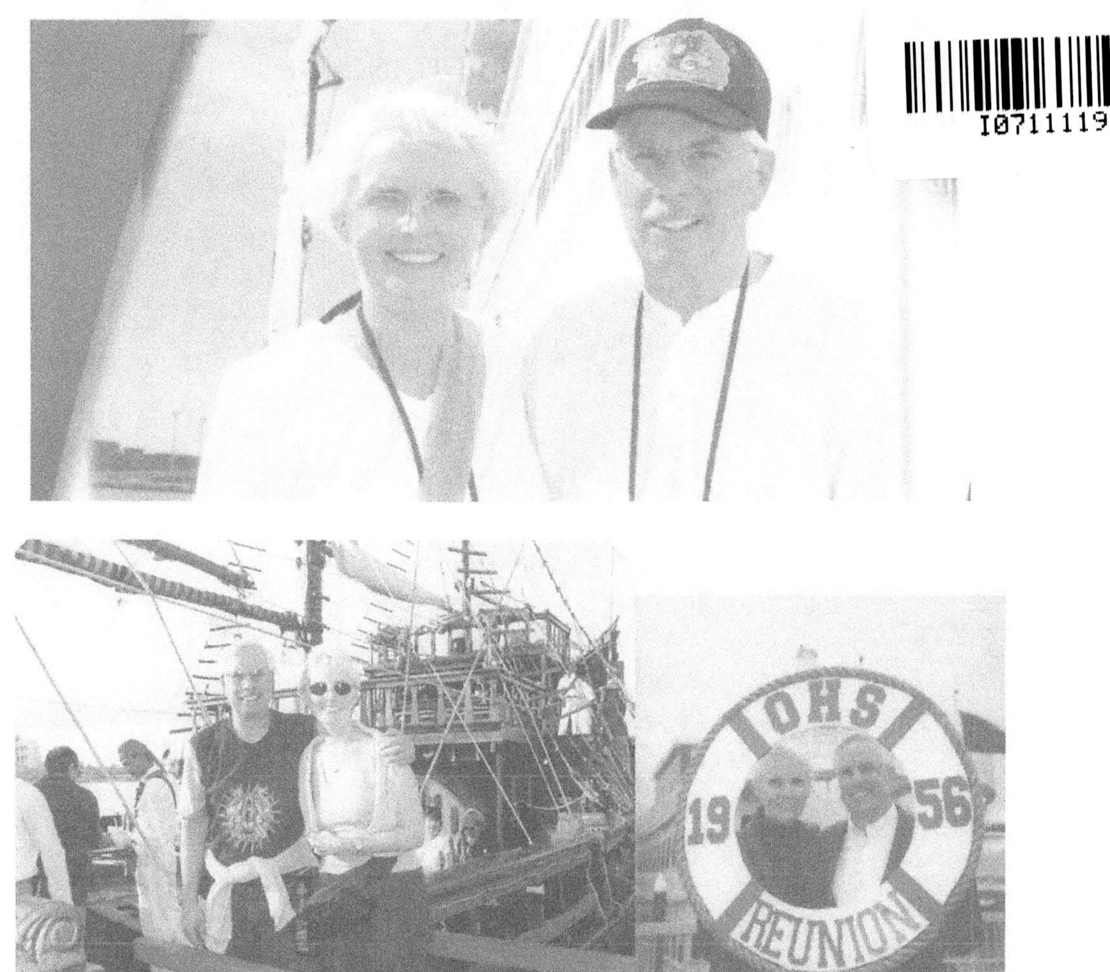

Kitty Wall

PAGE PUBLISHING, INC.
Conneaut Lake, PA

First originally published by Page Publishing 2020

ISBN 978-1-64701-170-3 (pbk)
ISBN 978-1-64701-171-0 (digital)

Printed in the United States of America

WORLDWIDE NEARLY FORTY-FOUR MILLION PEOPLE STRUGGLE WITH DEMENTIA, MONSTERS, SUCH AS PARKINSON, ALZHEIMER, HUNTINGTON, VASCULAR DISEASES, STROKE, DEPRESSION, CHRONIC DRUG USE, AND OTHERS.

This book is dedicated to my beloved husband, David Wall (1938–2015). David passed away at home with his family at his bedside. David was a wonderful husband and father, and I miss him very much.

EXACTLY THREE YEARS AFTER DAVID'S PASSING, HIS WISHES WERE FINALIZED. HIS CREMATED REMAINS WERE SET FREE DURING A PRIVATE CEREMONY PERFORMED ON TOP OF A SERENE MOUNTAIN OVERLOOKING BEAUTIFUL SYCAMORE CANYON NEAR SEDONA, ARIZONA.

MAY HIS SPIRIT FOREVER TRAVEL ON THE WINGS OF OUR LOVING THOUGHTS!

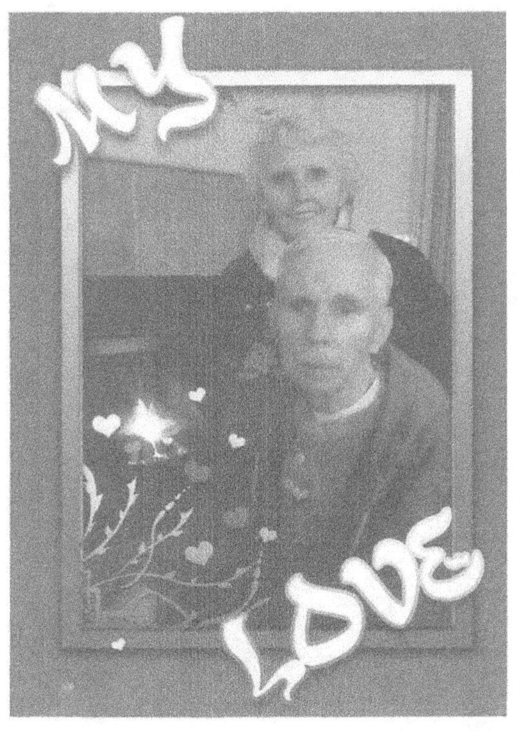

My Love

I also want to thank all the caring and loving caregivers. Special thanks to my daughter in law, and son who helped me through this time. Special thanks to my special friend, Tom H. Smith, author of *Dead Dog Barking*, who helped me put this together because it is hard to revisit most of these stressful memories.

Dear Reader,

I wrote this booklet guide after having personally cared for my husband, David. Together, we fought the DEMENTIA MONSTER for eight years. He did not know who I was for many of those years. Make no mistake, DEMENTIA is a terrible MONSTER that I want to help you confront, and yes, FIGHT AND HOPEFULLY CONQUER!

Many of you reading this have likely just been informed that you and your loved one will have to confront the same dementia monsters we did. No doubt the initial diagnosis will leave you grasping for answers and solutions. Believe me, I thoroughly realize that you are currently in the frustrated *"WHY US"* stage. This booklet contains our personal experiences and my hard-earned advice. I believe that if we had the enclosed information, it would have saved us a lot of agonies and frustration.

Unfortunately, during office visits, the medical doctors and staff have only a few minutes to discuss what you will be facing in the trying days, weeks, and possibly years ahead. But listen—with GOD'S GRACE, you must have faith that the scientists will soon discover a cure. My husband, David, and I fought an enduring battle. Unfortunately, now you too must face this MONSTROUS situation.

I pray the information within this guide will help you immensely! I genuinely wish I could take each of you by the hand and try to comfort everyone involved. Unfortunately, I can't do that! But hopefully, my over eight years of painful experiences will help you prevent the mistakes I made along the way. So please take the information I offer and let's battle this together.

With sincere love, truth, and understanding,
I AM THE WIDOW WALL (Ms. K. Wall)

Contents

My name is Kay Wall. I wrote this booklet with a determination to arm and inform everyone charged with caring for those diagnosed with dementia and related monstrous diseases. Unfortunately, I had to learn how best to try and confront the monster the medical industry calls DEMENTIA the hard way—on my own! Sadly, as of 2015, I have become the widow Wall. That is the year I lost my beloved husband, David Wall, to dementia and Parkinson disease. We fought these beasts for eight long and excruciating years. Hopefully, the enclosed information I am sharing will enable others to better confront the monster that they are about to engage.

I confess it was challenging writing about what my husband, David, and I went through with dementia and Parkinson disease because it brought back so many bad memories. I believe that is the reason there has never been a booklet quite like this one. Understandably, those that have encountered this struggle would prefer not to discuss the pain and suffering they endured during their battles. But with God's guidance, I felt the importance of sharing what I went thru in hopes of helping others.

My first recommendation is to *KNOW THE ENEMY*. So let's start with the facts. Officially dementia is a symptom of various diseases such as Parkinson, Alzheimer, Huntington, and several others, even drug abuse. There are medicines out there with side effects, so please check your medicines that you are taking. Officially, the definition of DEMENTIA is as follows: **loss of cognitive abilities, including memory, concentration, communication, planning, and abstract thinking, resulting from brain injury or from a disease such as Alzheimer disease or Parkinson disease. It is sometimes accompanied by emotional disturbance and personality changes.**

So DEMENTIA is a SYMPTOM of various diseases such as PARKINSON, ALZHEIMER, HUNTINGTON, VASCULAR DISEASES, STROKE, DEPRESSION, and CHRONIC DRUG USE. In reality, DEMENTIA is a common denominator symptom of various medical MONSTERS. Each dementia-related disease causes progressive damage to a different set of brain cells. Eventually, you will learn that dementia symptoms impact memory, the performance of daily activities, and communication abilities.

NOTE: To save space through this guide, I will use the word **DEMENTIA** instead of the long list of related diseases.

I must be upfront with you concerning what you are up against. You should know, in all honesty, that your journey is one of the most challenging experiences you hopefully will ever endure. The statistics reveal that the cases associated with dementia are in the tens of millions and rising every year. I'm sorry, but dementia is what it is—*A REAL MONSTER* to have to live with daily! However, I believe the information contained in this booklet will assist you in caring for your patient by at least knowing what to expect. It will also enable you to better provide pertinent information to your medical doctors and nurses about your patient or LOVED ONE.

In facing the facts concerning this horrific monster medically called DEMENTIA, there is NO cure YET! I truly realize this is a difficult statement to rationalize, but at least there is hope in the word "YET." Hopefully, someday soon it will be replaced by the phrase *"THANK GOD, THEY FOUND A CURE!"*

Since my husband passed away, there are promising new developments, which are in the works. In the meantime, there are some critical things you should understand that can help you prepare tremendously. I'm sorry, but speaking from many years of experience, you should expect and accept the fact that CONFUSION will come sooner or later with dementia. You must realize this and fully recognize and identify it for what it is. Through no fault of their own, the patient will have DISORIENTATION, UNCERTAINTY, PERPLEXITY, MISUNDERSTANDINGS, and MISPERCEPTIONS.

It is imperative to understand that the monster, DEMENTIA, eventually diminishes or destroys the patient's memories. One of the hardest things to endure is living with a loved one that doesn't know you anymore, SO BE PREPARED! Personally, I went through this nightmare of my dear husband, David, not knowing who I was for over eight painful years. So, therefore, I do indeed understand how difficult it is to take care of someone disabled by this horrible MONSTER.

Of course, it's painful, but I am going to reveal some of the personal things that we were involved with during David's illness. This is so you can perhaps benefit from our experiences. You may or may not go through the same involvements, but I include them, just in case you do. Hopefully, you will sooner or later appreciate and utilize my advice. Also, I have included vendors and resources that I found to be recommendable.

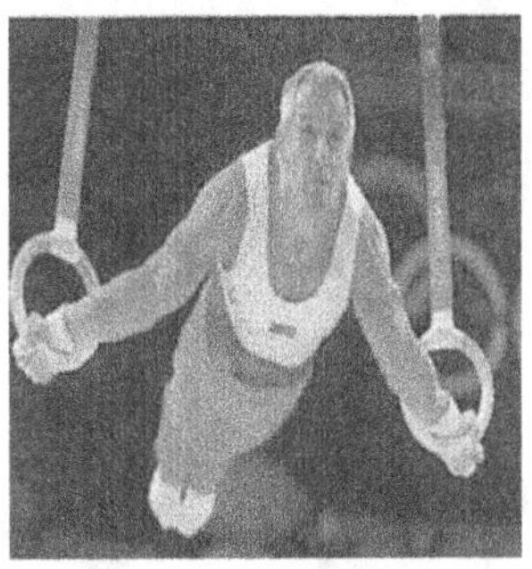

Olympic Rings

In David's youth, he participated in wrestling and gymnastics. He was even at the Olympic qualifying level. It's odd, but David was told during the time he competed that people involved in gymnastics were prone to get Parkinson disease. He thought it was because of the pressure on gymnast's nerves on the Olympic rings.

Throughout our marriage, David and I were very much in love, and we shared the same goals in life. He was a mechanical engineer in the space program, and I was in the accounting field. Like many others, we worked very hard to survive and to prepare for taking care of ourselves in retirement. However, later, as his wife, I noticed he began having problems with his math and reading and short-term memory loss. Upon examination, our primary doctor referred us to a neurologist. I made an appointment with a neurologist, and she performed a memory test and MRI. The results showed no signs of Alzheimer disease. However, the neurologist referred us to a sleep apnea department because of David's loud snoring. The neurologist told us sleep apnea could cause dementia because he wasn't getting enough sleep.

(Continuous Positive Airway Pressure)
(SOURCES LISTED IN THE BACK OF BOOKLET)

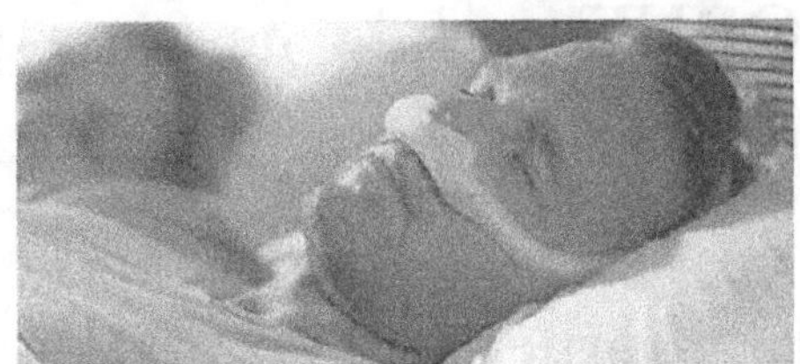

"Continuous positive airway pressure is a form of positive airway pressure ventilator, which applies mild air pressure on a continuous basis to keep the airways continuously open in people who can breathe spontaneously on their own" (Wikipedia).

The neurologist wanted us to come back in six months to do another memory test on him. The sleep apnea department tested him, and he showed definite for SLEEP APNEA. We started him on the CPAP (*continuous positive airway pressure*) for sleep apnea treatment. The CPAP machine helped get oxygen to his brain while David was sleeping and better enables rest.

About a month later, David came into the kitchen and asked me if I was his wife. He also exclaimed that he felt that he had died and then came back to life. It was at that point that I knew I had to get some help. David began having trouble adjusting to the CPAP. Therefore, I called the sleep apnea department, and they referred me to the psychologist department. So I made an appointment with a psychologist to deal with his confusion. The psychologist felt he had Parkinson disease because of David's lack of facial expressions, which he called **STONE FACE,** also called **PARKINSON MASK** and **POKER FACE.** They also did some memory test there, but he tested well at that time.

LEGAL SERVICES RECOMMENDED

(SOURCES LISTED IN THE BACK OF BOOKLET)

It was then David and I agreed that we needed to do a **DURABLE POWER OF ATTORNEY** while he was still capable, which was extremely important! That legal document gave me the authority to manage David's property.

(PLEASE NOTE: The attorney will do ONLY ONE original and make copies of that original. So put the original in a secure place, such as a safe deposit box at the bank. The attorney will have at his office a copy only.)

Of course, it's essential that an attorney does the will because it might be challenged later. Therefore, the will should be reviewed every couple of years.

I recommend you consult with experts at Medicaid planning, nursing home rights, Medicare, guardianship, elder abuse, Social Security, and estate planning such as National Academy of Elder Law Attorneys and National Elder Law Foundation. Now, even though you have a LIVING TRUST, it's still important to have a will because it's impossible to put all your assets into a Trust.

Please BEWARE: general **POWER OF ATTORNEY** ends when a person becomes mentally incapable because of sickness or injury to handle his or her own affairs. However, a **DURABLE POWER OF ATTORNEY** does not stop in these circumstances, and it doesn't expire until death.

Please note: All originals need to be secured in a safe place. I suggest a bank safe deposit or a safe at home.

Contact by entering naela.org and nelf.org for certifying practitioners of elderly and special-needs law.

HOME SECURITY SYSTEM/ DEVICES AND EQUIPMENT

(SOURCES LISTED IN BACK OF BOOKLET)

Now, in our case several years after being tested every year, the neurologist and psychologist determined David had dementia and Parkinson. Eventually, we took him off the CPAP machine because it was no longer doing him any good. Also, the doctors had his driver's license revoked, as a safety precaution.

At that time, the psychologist instructed me to remove dangerous items such as knives, matches, power tools, electric gadgets. Also, and most importantly, guns kept in the house should have safety locks or else eliminate them altogether. The psychologist instructed me if my husband got violent to please notify him.

Eventually, David began to know me less and less. Therefore, for his safety, I had a security system (ADT) installed in our home and an alarm system attached to our bedroom doors that I could hear him get up in the middle of the night. Nevertheless, he did run away three times, but thankfully I was able to quickly locate him.

I also discovered that our sheriff department had a volunteer program for helping people with dementia. I called them, and a sheriff came to our house and attached a GPS device to David's wrist. They also took a photo of him, and I kept one of him too. Afterward, the sheriff's officer came out once a month to change the GPS battery. This worked out well. I told David that this was for his safety, and he accepted it; he had to be watched twenty-four hours a day.

Here are three points I discovered that very much pertain:

1. *A good rule to follow is to let people do for themselves if they get frustrated, and then assist them.*
2. *Keep them independent for as long as possible and safe always.*
3. *Don't rush them.*

(SOURCES LISTED IN BACK OF BOOKLET)

Eventually, our primary doctor referred us to Social Services. A Social Services nurse came out and evaluated our medical needs and safety in our home. She prescribed a chair/handrail for the shower and a handrail by the toilet for safety. She referred me to a medical supply store that accepted Medicare for renting a wheelchair and a walker.

David also needed a physical therapist and a speech therapist, and they came out to our house four times in total. They helped him with physical exercises and for his speaking. We did these workouts every day. This enabled him in walking and assisted him to get out of a chair. Eventually, I realized that I needed help with lifting David because I was raising his dead weight, and it was just getting too strenuous for me.

LONG-TERM CARE INSURANCE

(SOURCES LISTED IN BACK OF BOOKLET)

We were very fortunate to have long-term care insurance. Without it, I don't know what we would have done financially. Long-term care insurance is insurance usually purchased before a person becomes ill. It helps cover long-term care requirements such as nursing homes, residential or assisted care homes, and adult day care. I informed our long-term care insurance that my husband, David, had dementia and Parkinson and that I needed a caregiver in my home. They instructed me to call several caregiver providers. Caregiver providers will come out to your home and let you know their policies, cost, etc. You should tell them that you have long-term care insurance and they are going to have to bill insurance. Also, they need to know what kind of care is required and how many hours and days you need a caregiver. I also furnished a copy of my scheduled itemized daily list of the duties for the caregivers. I provided them my long-term care insurance's name, address, phone number, and policy number so they can invoice/bill them. I had two caregiver providers in case one couldn't work that day. I phoned my long-term care insurance and gave them the two caregiver providers' names, address, phone numbers, and contact person.

(SOURCES LISTED IN BACK OF BOOKLET)

In the beginning, we had caregivers part-time. Then later on, it became seven days per week from 9:00 a.m. to 5:00 p.m. Now, from my experience, I recommend having a schedule itemized daily list for the caregivers. This will help maintain regular daily organization. I cannot stress enough the importance of quality CAREGIVING for your loved one. Remember, you are their primary CAREGIVER, but you need others as well.

Therefore, I will offer you some valuable advice on how best to work with professional caregivers. Most importantly, you need to set the work standards and the level of excellence you expect for your loved one. Otherwise, it is customary for people to not do any more than they must. So you must let caregivers know exactly what needs to be done and when. Anything else is unfair to your loved one and to you! So you need a **CAREGIVER SCHEDULE**—*AND MAINTAIN AND ENFORCE IT TWENTY-FOUR HOURS EVERY DAY.*

The caregiver will use this list/schedule and check items off when the care is given.

Note: Attached is a sample of a scheduled itemized daily list. You need to develop your own scheduled itemized daily list.

One such item is noted when the caregiver arrives in the morning, and if my husband, David, were awake, we would massage his legs and gently exercise them while he was in bed. If he were sleeping, we would wait until he is fully awake so that his walking would be more stable. It's also important to remember he needs to be in a happy environment as much as possible.

DISPOSAL UNDERGARMENT

(SOURCES LISTED IN BACK OF BOOKLET)

When David was awake, we would remove all his wet clothes and overnight disposable underwear.

NOTE: HYGIENE IS VERY IMPORTANT!

So depending on the patient's mood, they should be asked if they want a shower, a tub bath, or a sponge.

Thankfully, I discovered dressing my husband, David, in the bathroom while positioned on the toilet; it was much more comfortable with him and us. Also, pants with elastic waistbands made putting his clothes on easier.

Schedule caregivers to prepare breakfasts. Also give supplements orally or mash them into orange juice, hot cereal, or applesauce. Caregivers should keep patient active during the day and often check to see if the bathroom is needed. Schedule caregivers to fix lunch and maintain patient's activeness during the rest of the day and check on bathroom needs. Later, in the day, they changed his clothes and disposable underwear needed.

I recommend using a TRANSFER BENCH SWIVEL, SLIDES IN AND OUT OF SHOWER OR TUB, for patient's easy access and for safety. **IMPORTANT: WHEN YOU ORDER YOU WILL NEED SIZE OF SHOWER OR TUB.**

Contact amazon.com by entering transfer bench swivel, slides in and out of shower or tub.

I also recommend showering the patient at least twice a week if you can or sponge baths every day. **DEPENDING ON THE PATIENTS MOOD, I WOULD ASK THEM IF THEY WANT A SHOWER.** Sometimes, patients may need to be told that they need a shower. The important thing is to create a friendly, not a FORCED situation.

(WETTING AND SOILING)

Incontinence issues need to be discussed with your doctor—AS WITH everything concerning patient care. Check often to see if the patient needs to be taken to the bathroom frequently. I recommend TENA (*light and heavy*) incontinence pads for men/women under the patient's clothing for added protection. Later, you will need DAY and OVERNIGHT disposable underwear protection. *Keep track of how often the patient urinates, and record on the caregivers' schedule.*

I recommend Tranquility (brand) day and overnight disposable absorbent underwear. Contact by entering one of these sites for Tranquility incontinence products:

www.nationalincontinence.com.www.IncontinenceProductsPlus.com
www.walmart.com
www.tranquilityproducts.com.

- Your primary doctor should refer you to social workers for social and emotional issues, as well as living situations for safety needs. The social worker also should refer you to a physical therapist to improve patient mobility and safety. They should recommend a speech therapist if needed.

- GPS (global positioning system): GPS, if it is available in your area, is for tracking/locating your patient AT ALL TIMES from the air and ground. You must be prepared for when your patient WANDERS! Check with your local sheriff department, for the wrist-worn version. *Our GPS was a volunteer program furnished by the local sheriff department.*

- ADT SYSTEM: Install a quality security system. ADT system is what we used.

- Keep patient active during the day because it helps them from wandering in the middle of the night.

- I discovered that changing a patient's clothes is much more accessible while they are positioned on the toilet.

- Be aware that when dementia and Parkinson disease progress, the patient's muscles will stiffen. Therefore, it becomes difficult for your patient to get out of a chair/bed. They also can become stooped over and develop a shuffling walk. Thus, a caregiver needs to always be by the patient's side AT ALL TIMES!

- While walking the patient, always have them take the caregiver's arm. That arm should be held close to the caregiver's body to maintain balance for both patient and caregiver.

- When lifting, try to always avoid leaning forward or bending over. You should only bend at the knees, not at the waist. If you raise a person, do it from under the armpits to avoid injuring the patient.

- When a patient falls, try not to get upset, and gently calm them down. Ask them if they can get themselves up. If they are not able to get up, seek assistance or call 911—SAVE your back!

- The psychologist instructed me to remove dangerous items such as knives, matches, power tools, electric gadgets, and guns kept in the house should have a safety lock or get rid of them.

- Use plastic utensils, plate, and cup when serving meals.

- Don't leave medicines where the patient can access

- AARP (October 2, 2017, bulletin), laundry detergent pods, liquid packets, and laundry packets (dementia patients are eating them and dying). Therefore, remove pods, packets, and detergents from the patient's access.

- Naturally, always make sure the patient's car door is locked while transporting.

- Eliminate clutter in the house and rugs that the patient can slip on.

- BED ALARM WITH BED PAD OR FLOORMAT ALARM: I also strongly advise wireless (cord-free) bed alarm with bed pad or floormat alarm with a wireless pager to let you know they are getting out of bed. This also helps the patient from wandering and falling.
  Contact amazon.com by entering an alarm bed pad or floormat alarm.

- WHEELCHAIR ALARM SYSTEM: I strongly advise attaching an alarm system on the patient's wheelchair to let you know they are getting out of the chair.
  Contact: amazon.com by entering wheelchair alarm.

- DOORS and WINDOWS ALARMS: I recommend installing door and window alarms if needed. This also helps the patient from wandering away.

- MONITOR: Put a monitor in the bedroom to let you know if the patient gets out of bed while you are somewhere else in the house. Contact: amazon.com by entering "BABY MONITORS FOR THE BEDROOM."
- STANDARD HOSPITAL BEDS: Standard hospital beds help the caregivers with putting the patient in and out of bed safely (see rent, Medicare part B). Contact by entering www.medicare.gov.

I HOPE YOU GET THESE SECURITY/SAFETY DEVICES BECAUSE I REMEMBER SO MANY NIGHTS NOT GETTING ANY SLEEP. YOU NEED TO GET YOUR REST SO YOU WILL BE ABLE TO TAKE CARE OF YOUR PATIENT AND ALSO FOR YOUR HEALTH.

Another problem to watch out for is sundowning, also known as (sundowner syndrome). It isn't a disease but a group of symptoms that occur in the late afternoon or early evening. The patient can become confused, disoriented, agitated, angry, depressed, restless, paranoid, and moody in the late afternoon hours. Other behaviors to look out for are rocking, crying, pacing, hiding things, acting out violently, and wandering. The patient may even experience hallucinations. So keep the evening calm and turn the lights on in the afternoon, before dark. Also, discourage daytime napping, but encourage day exercises.

Limit the patient's caffeine intake and sugar in the evening. In the evening, you can even play soothing music before the patient goes to bed. Sometimes my husband had issues with sundowning. My husband, David, was a very gentle and kind man, but the monster dementia made him agitated sometimes, and a caregiver would get clobbered. One time I got slugged in the stomach, but I knew that it wasn't my David; it was the dementia. You need to know that your loved one isn't entirely there mentally anymore, and that's one of the most challenging problems to cope with.

NOTE: I hope you noticed by now with the information I provided so far that it's critical not to ignite your patient's agitation fuse. Otherwise, any sign of your agitation is likely to produce a temper explosion.

It's human nature for every action to produce a reaction. Therefore, try to always have this in mind. A caregiver's anger doesn't battle the monster dementia; it helps the monster progress against the patient. My own observation is that the frustration a patient exhibits is due to their being trapped in confusion and their inability to overcome the mental hold the monster dementia has on them.

Sundowning/sundowner syndrome needs to be discussed with your doctor, AS WITH everything concerning patient care. In David's case, my primary doctor prescribed calming medicine, and it helped to calm him down.

This helped with his stiffness (Parkinson) and relaxed his muscles at night for better sleep. Before leaving, I scheduled the caregiver to put on the patient's overnight disposal underwear and pajamas. I prepared our dinner and changed his overnight disposal underwear if it was wet. Now, to prepare him for sleep, I would give patient nonhabit natural sleep tape on his tongue at night or mash a nonhabit sleep pill into patient's food/drink.

- MOST IMPORTANTLY IS GIVING THEM LOVE AND KEEPING THEM HAPPY.
- You also need to humor them. Provide a happy environment always.
- Always, keep them active if you can and of course safe.
- Also, be prepared for dementia to worsen!

For more information regarding sundowning/sundowner syndrome: Contact by entering http://www.carinq.com and http://wwwmayoclinic.org

- NEWSPAPERS/BOOKS: Read to the patient and have them read back to you (ask them questions).
- FAMILY PICTURES: Ask them, "Who is this?"
- PUZZLES: Example: USA Map Wooden Puzzle of the United States of America by Melissa and Doug. Contact amazon.com by entering "US puzzle map game."
- BLOCK PUZZLE: Example: Wooden Preschool Shape Puzzle by Gibber and Mum. Contact amazon.com by entering "kids learning blocks."
- CARD GAMES: Example: Go Fish card game by the Peaceable Kingdom. Contact amazon.com by entering "go fish card game for kids."
- GAMES: Example: Campbell's Crossword Game; it helps the patient put words together.
  Contact amazon.com by entering "Campbell's alphabet dice game."
- SMALL EXERCISE BIKE: I can recommend an exercise bike made by Eva medical pedal exerciser with chrome frame (fully assembled) arm exerciser and leg pedal cycle to chair and put feet in pedals.
  Contact amazon.com by entering "EVA PEDAL EXERCISER."
- WALK OR USE WHEELCHAIR: Take patient for a walk or wheelchair them around the neighborhood but always attended by a caregiver.
- TV: I recommend watching TV for only two hours (no violent or sad shows). Keep them active as much as you can during the day. This will help the patient from wandering around at night and for you to get rest too.
- MUSIC: Calm, soothing, NOT head-banging, chaotic music type.

- SENIOR CENTERS: Some senior centers have activities for people with dementia/Parkinson.
  Contact senior centers within your local area.
- PHYSICAL THERAPY EXERCISES: Physical therapy exercises will help the patient with walking. These exercises are essential because it strengthens their leg muscles for walking and sitting and enables standing. This also reduces agitation, helps them to sleep instead of wandering, prevents depression, and improves self-esteem. *Medicare pays for a certain number of physical therapist visits.*

COPING AND BEING ACTIVE YOURSELF

Now, as I stated in the beginning, I want to talk about your having to care for your patient. You must realize dementia and Parkinson disease are things NONE of us asked to be part of. The information I am furnishing you was gathered over eight years of my life. That is the same number of years that a PhD spends learning their profession. Yet they did not have to deal with their loved ones going through dementia and Parkinson disease on a 24/7 basis. So here are my suggestions on how best to survive this ordeal (not in any specific order):

- Parkinson and Alzheimer support groups
- Keeping busy
- Gym or exercise at home
- School (take some classes)
- Painting and crafts
- Photography
- Senior club
- Household chores
- Bills/finance
- Do things that make you and your patient happy
- Church
- Take one day at a time

- ADULT WALKER DEVICES: Various types. Folding, nonfolding, wheeled, etc. Rent through MEDICARE PART B.
  Contact www.medicare.gov.
- HURRICANE CANE by Hurry Cane Company
  Contact amazon.com and enters the words **"HURRICANE CANE."**
- TRAVEL WHEELCHAIR: They are lighter to handle and transport.
- Rent through MEDICARE PART B.
  Contact www.medicare.gov.
- WHEELCHAIR: Later on, as the disease progresses, you will need a better wheelchair because your patient will be sitting in them more. Rent through MEDICARE PART B.
  Contact www.medicare.gov.
- CUSHION PADS FOR WHEELCHAIR: I recommend air/water cushion, gel pads, and foam pads for wheelchair to prevent pressure sores.
  Contact amazon.com and enter the words **"WHEELCHAIR AIR CUSHION."**
- RECLINER CHAIR: I recommend a recliner chair that lifts the patient. Rent them through MEDICARE PART B.
  Contact www.medicare.gov.
- SHOWER/TUB TRANSFER BENCH: I stress having a shower/tub transfer bench that swivels, slides in and out of shower or tub.
  Contact amazon.com and enter the words **"TRANSFER BENCH THAT SWIVELS, SLIDES IN AND OUT OF SHOWER AND TUB."**

Important: you will need to measure your shower/tub before ordering.

- SHOWER HANDRAILS: Install sturdy shower handrails. Contact amazon.com and enter the words **"SHOWER HANDRAILS."**
- HANDRAIL NEAR TOILET: Install sturdy HAND BAR close to the toilet. Contact amazon.com and enter the words: **"TOILET HANDRAILS."**
- TOILET SEAT RISER: To help patient rise off the toilet seat. Contact amazon.com and enter the words **"TOILET SEAT RISER."**
- ADDED (soft) TOILET SEATS: Padded soft toilet seats are more comfortable for the person who must sit for long periods of time. Contact amazon.com and enter the words **"PADDED SOFT TOILET SEATS."**
- ALTERNATING PRESSURE MATTRESS by Vive—includes electric pump and mattress pad—inflatable bed pad for pressure ulcer and pressure sore treatment fits standard hospital beds. This is what we used, and it really helped prevent pressure sores. Contact amazon.com enter the words **"PRESSURE MATTRESS BY VIVE."**
- CALMOSEPTINE OINTMENT (*Long-Lasting Protection*): It protects and helps heal skin irritations caused by incontinence of urine or diarrhea and diaper rash, etc.: *"This also helped prevent and heal pressure sores."* Contact amazon.com and enter the words **"CALMOSEPTINE OINTMENT."**
- TRANQUILITY (brand) INCONTINENCE PRODUCTS PREMIUM OVERNIGHT DISPOSABLE ABSORBENT UNDERWEAR (**this holds over a quart**): This helped prevent soiling the bed and also having to change the bedding as often.

- TRANQUILITY INCONTINENCE PRODUCTS **DAY UNDERWEAR** TOO.
- The ample, full-waist panel provides a more proportioned fit. (Pull-on style with tearaway side seams allow for easy removal.)
Contact www.IncontinenceProductsPlus.com
- DISPOSAL MEDICAL GLOVES: Used for changing underwear, soiled clothes, bedding, and cleaning patient, etc.
Contact amazon.com by entering **"disposal medical gloves"** (also available at drugstores).
- SUREGUARD (brand) MATTRESS PROTECTOR: This product is to protect against bedwetting, perspiration, liquids, dust mites, 100 percent allergens, bacteria, mildew, and mold. (Also, I would put a fitted sheet over the mattress protector if needed.)
Contact amazon.com by entering "PROTECTIVE PAD FOR MATTRESS."

This is a sample: A new daily CAREGIVER SCHEDULE was provided each day.

NOTE: BY HAVING A SCHEDULE FOR CAREGIVERS, THE PATIENT WILL GET THE RIGHT CARE THAT IS NEEDED. You will need to develop your own schedule!

CAREGIVERS DO NOT GIVE MEDICINES—YOU HAVE TO TRAIN EACH CAREGIVERS
- In an emergency: Please call me at ____.
- Bathroom every two hours (because he forgets).
- Stay close to the patient when they are walking.
- Report and record BEHAVIORAL problems.
- Record bowel movements on this schedule: How many daily? ____

CIRCLE MOVEMENT (small, medium, large)
- How many times did they urinate? ____
  Check off or line out what has been done.

MORNING: (HAPPY ENVIRONMENT)
- Needs to wake up by himself if possible because the patient gets confused.
- Massage and exercise patient's legs gently.
- Take wet clothes off and put in bag/basket for laundry.
- Shower or sponge bath (always dry out shower) every Sat. and Wed.

Depending on mood, ask them if they want a shower.

- Wet towels always put in bag/basket for laundry.
- Put the patient's clothes on and their disposal underwear with insert.
- If bedsheets are wet, *take protector pad and sheet off the bed and put in bag/basket for laundry.*

MORNING:

- Wash wet sheets separate from other clothes.
- Install a clean protector pad and sheet on the bed.

BREAKFAST (plastic fork, spoon, and cup only for safety)

- Orange juice with hemp oil, fish oil, coconut oil, vitamin E, and stool softener (puncture hole in the capsule and squeeze into orange juice and stir it up.)
- One banana.
- Dry or hot cereal milk/water (plastic bowl and spoon). Hot cereals, stir in BARLEAN'S extra-virgin coconut oil.

CHECK OFF OR LINE OUT WHAT HAS BEEN DONE

- Two pieces of toast (with jam/butter on sourer dough or raisin bread). When giving medicines, I would crush tablets and put in apple-sauce or orange juice. Always, check with a doctor about how to give medications.
- Wash dishes.
- Brush teeth.
- Read the morning paper and have the patient read it back.

LUNCH: (examples)

- Sandwich or soup with crackers and V8 Juice or VA Splash.

- Wash dishes.
- After lunch, give the patient Gatorade and lots of water.

SNACKS: (examples)
- I provided any of these: yogurt, peanut butter crackers, Quaker bars, ice cream, or fruit.

EXERCISES:
- Bike for legs and arms (morning and afternoon), with or without music.
- Exercises use a dining room chair.
- Physical therapy exercises.
- Morning walk or wheelchair with caregiver (not in the heat).

KEEP PATIENT ACTIVE:
- TV, two hours (nonviolent and sad movies). No TV two hours before bedtime.
- Plays catch with the patient (ball).
- Construct puzzles with the patient—I recommend USA Map Wooden Puzzle of United States of America.
- Play games with the patient—I recommend Campbell Soup game.
- Color (with a coloring book) with the patient.
- On a writing tablet, have the patient write words, numbers, or draw something.

NOTE: *KEEPING PATIENT ACTIVE DURING THE DAY HELPS PREVENTS THEM FROM WANDERING AROUND AT NIGHT.*

HOUSEWORK ON WEDNESDAY AND SATURDAY: WHATEVER NEEDS TO BE CLEANED?

- Check off or line out what has been done (this really helped the caregiver and me).
- BEFORE CAREGIVERS LEAVE, THEY WOULD PUT ON HIS PAJAMAS and OVERNIGHT DISPOSAL ABSORBENT UNDERWEAR.

I would fix my patient's dinner, change his overnight disposal absorbent underwear if needed, and put a sleeping pill in his drink or food. This helped him to sleep and relax his muscles.

NOTE: BY HAVING A SCHEDULE FOR CAREGIVERS, THE PATIENT WILL GET THE RIGHT CARE THAT IS NEEDED.

This information is given to our caregivers in case of emergency—PLEASE develop your own!

NAME OF CONTACTS/PHONE NUMBER: ___________________

NAME (PATIENT): ___________________

ADDRESS: ___________________

DATE OF BIRTH: ___________________

PRIMARY INSURANCE: ___________________

PRIMARY DOCTOR NAME AND PHONE NUMBER: ___________

MEDICAL ISSUES: Dementia and Parkinson ___________________

LIST OF PATIENT'S MEDICINES THEY ARE TAKING:

___________________   ___________________

___________________   ___________________

___________________   ___________________

***ALLERGIC TO THESE MEDICATIONS:**

* ___________________

* ___________________

* ___________________

In David's case, his dementia problem progressed more and more rapidly, and eventually, he needed two caregivers, and I was his second caregiver. Before dementia, David weighed 175 pounds, and his height was five feet and eight inches. Gradually David's dementia worsened, and he was not able to eat anymore; he eventually weighed only eighty-five pounds, and his height dropped to five feet and one inch in this debilitating condition.

So now I'm going to talk to you about something many of you might not know much about; it's called HOSPICE; it's specialized care. I phoned a HOSPICE service, and a representative and nurse came out to evaluate David. HOSPICE told me that we couldn't do any more for him and not to force-feed him because it could cause more pain for him. He needed to be in HOSPICE. Also, HOSPICE instructed me to find a funeral home of our choice. Beware that hospice care does not include a nurse in your home 24/7. While on HOSPICE, we kept our own caregivers and kept in contact with HOSPICE. However, HOSPICE has nurses and doctors on call 24/7. While he was in hospice, he still wouldn't eat, and he had a hard time breathing. Hospice provided strong pain meds to calm him down and other medicines.

Hospice providers furnish a no-cost emergency treatment package, and they will instruct usage.

Also, note pharmacy supplies and medications will be delivered to your home from only the sources that the HOSPICE provider uses.

CAUTION: *BEWARE THAT STRONG PAIN MEDS ARE IN THIS PACKAGE AND MUST BE REFRIGERATED THEREFORE SAFEGUARD.*

I informed HOSPICE the name of the funeral home and who to talk to. David was in HOSPICE for just one week before he passed away. When they pass at home, HOSPICE will remove them from their home. I informed the funeral home that David had passed away, and HOSPICE will be contacting them. The funeral home I chose also had a grieving assistant. The HOSPICE of your choice should also provide in-home chaplain counseling services as needed.

Hospice care is covered by Medicare in all states and by Medicaid in most states, as well as by most insurance plans and health maintenance organizations (HMOs). However, you should understand that while in HOSPICE, you cannot receive any medical assistant services from any other source other than the HOSPICE source you're contracted with. Please note if the patient requires hospital-type services, they will need to get off the HOSPICE program until those services are no longer involved. However, HOSPICE CAN BE REINSTATED.

Hospice only provides services to patients at their resident/home or assistant living / nursing home location and inpatient residential centers and hospitals with hospice care options. However, VERY FEW HOSPITALS OFFER HOSPICE CARE.

NOTE: *Insurance companies dread patients getting on and off hospice because it is difficult to determine who is responsible for paying. Sometimes it's difficult getting back on hospice, AND YOU MAYBE BILLED IN THE PROCESS.*

Some hospice providers have their own inpatient facilities. Also note pharmacy supply and medications will only be covered and delivered to your home from ONLY the sources that particular HOSPICE pharmacy sources. When a patient passes away in their home, HOSPICE will provide removal from their home. The funeral home services have to be set up by you. The funeral home you choose should have grief assistance. Then you contact hospice, and they will take the patient's body to the funeral home of your choice. The hospice of your choice should also provide in-home chaplain counseling services weekly or as needed. There is a misconception concerning hospice care. It is not always a death sentence; there are exceptions to that rule.

CASE IN POINT: I have a close friend diagnosed with bladder cancer in 2011. He was passing more blood than urine, and his family doctor placed him in HOSPICE care at that time. Within a few months receiving in-home hospice care and fervent prayer, he completely recovered and for six years now has been entirely in remission.

How hospice works / Medicare.gov:
Learn how hospice works, about team providers, where to get help, how long care lasts, how to find a provider, and when to stop.
Contact by entering www.medicare.gov.

In-Home Hospice Services:
Phone: 844-668-9804
Contact by entering www.Hospice.CareinHomes.com.

KINDRED HOSPICE CO.:
Comfort and support at home.
Phone: 866-509-4146
Contact by entering www.qo.kindred.com/Hospice-Care.

AMBERCARE CO.:
Offers hospice care—in the home.
Phone: 877-861-0060
Contact by entering www.ambercare.com/hospice-care.

MAYO CLINIC CO.:
Will explain who's involved in hospice care.
Contact by entering www.mayoclinic.org/healthy.

Please realize these plans are expensive but can be a really GREAT financial help. The cost depends on your age, so please research those carefully before you invest.

We decided on purchasing long-term care insurance because we had assets and our family did not live close by to help. We recognized we would need help if one of us became unable to assist. Looking back, long-term care insurance was the best investment that we made. I don't know how we would have survived without it financially. Before my husband, David, was diagnosed, we invested in Bankers' long-term care insurance. They really helped me afford caregivers to help take care of my husband suffering from dementia and Parkinson.

NOTE: It is possible to purchase long-term care insurance after diagnosis. However, of course, the cost is much more expensive.

LONG-TERM CARE INSURANCE:

Contact Bankers Life and Casualty Co., Policy Benefits Dept., PO Box 1902, Carmel, IN 46082-1935

Phone: 800-621-3724 or 800-654-3072

For additional information about dementia and Parkinson.
Enter https://en.wikipedia.org/wiki/Dementia. **It's a free encyclopedia.**

These are excellent books on helping you slay these MONSTERS.

***THE 36-HOUR DAY*, FIFTH EDITION**
Published 2012
By Nancy L. Mace, MA, and Peter V. Rabins, MD, MPH

***THE 36-HOUR DAY*, SIXTH EDITION**
Published 2017
By Nancy L. Mace, MA, and Peter V. Rabins, MD, MPH

***HOW TO CARE FOR AGING PARENTS*, THIRD EDITION**
Published 2014
By Virginia Morris

Alzheimer Association

225 N. Michigan Ave. Floor 17 Chicago, IL 60601-7633

Phone: 800-272-3900

This site contains information about the organization, research, and care. It will connect you to your local chapter websites.

Contact by entering www.alz.org.

American Parkinson Disease Association (APDA)

This is an organization that gives patient and family support.

Contact by entering www.apdaparkinson.org.

National Institute on Aging's Alzheimer Disease Education and Research (ADEAR)

This site discusses current research and care strategies and also lists (with the web links) the Alzheimer Research Center.

Contact by entering www.nia.nih.gov/Alzheimer/AlzheimersInformation/About.org).

Leading Age

A nonprofit agency this has information about nursing homes, adult day care, assisted living, and other resources.

Contact by entering www.aahsa.org.

The National Consumer Voice for Quality Long-Term Care (nonprofit organization)

The National Consumer Voice for Quality Long-Term Care has information about nursing home advocacy. They also have a valuable document titled **"A Resident's Rights in Nursing Homes."** It covers the resident's rights in assisted living centers, board and care, and in-home and community care. It also lists the nursing home ombudspersons by state.
Contact by entering www.theconsumervoice.org.

ALWAYS USE THIS SITE TO COMPARE A SPECIFIC NURSING HOME WITH OTHER FACILITIES:
Contact by entering www.medicare.gov/nhcompare/home.asp.

Centers for Medicare and Medicaid Services
7500 Security Blvd., Baltimore, MD 21244-1850
Phone: 800-633-4227
Furnishes information about coverage and about Medicare Advantage programs. Medicare Part B pays for durable medical supplies, and wheelchairs. Medicare Part D is a prescription drug plan.
Contact by entering www.medicare.gov.

Medicaid
This federal website has state-by-state Medicaid information; this will direct you to your local Medicaid offices.
Contact by entering www.medicaid.gov.

John Hopkins Memory and Alzheimer Center
It furnishes videos reviewing how to deal with and care for a person with dementia.
Contact by entering www.hopkinsmedicine.org/dementia_virtual_support_group).

NATIONAL LONG-TERM CARE OMBUDSMAN RESOURCE 202 CENTER is an organization.

(Ombudsman is a government official or an employee who investigates complaints and tries to deal with them).

Phone: 202-332-2275

This website will direct you to a local ombudsman. They can find you nursing homes, assisted living centers, and other long-term care facilities and apprise you of your rights and help resolve conflicts with a facility.

Contact by entering <u>ltcombudsman.org</u>.

AARP (American Association of Retired Persons)

Provides information on caregiving, financial, and legal matters.

Phone: 888-687-2277

Contact by entering www.aarp.org.

Family Caregiver Alliance (nonprofit organization)

Provides useful information in caring for an elderly person.

Phone: 800-445-8106

Benefits Checkup (organization)

Information about prescription drug programs that can save money.

Contact by entering www.benefitscheckup.org.

by K. Wall

They come in all different sizes.
They can be vibrant, distinguish, and stand out among others.
They can be social climbers.
They can be hard to handle.
They can be a wallflower.
They can hurt others.
They can be expensive to others.
They need special attention.
They also attend many celebrations.
They can make people happy or sad.
They can be very popular with others.
They have several names.
They also come in different colors.
They can wilt and die.
So all—all roses could be people

by K. Wall

Life is just like a lily
Tall, strong, and vibrant beauty.
As the days go by, the vibrant beauty turns in to a faded soften complex beauty.
As the days go by, more it turns in to an everlasting inner beauty.
As the days go by, more the inner lasting beauty waits to be awakened when it is called upon.

Kitty Wall was born in Battle Creek, Michigan, but raised in Glendale, California. She had no siblings, so she was a brat. But she had a great childhood. She married and had three children, two boys and a girl. Unfortunately, the marriage ended. She went to school and learned accounting. So on her own, she raised her children. To this day, doing things with her children was the most enjoyable time in her life.

After her children grew up, she met David and fell in love. They had the same goals in life. They had a great life. She lost her best friend David and her mother.

She has three grandchildren and four great-grandchildren. She is presently living in Arizona with her two dogs, Glory and Dingo; two cats, Sugar and Spice; and a sun conure bird named Sunshine. She is surrounded by family and enjoying life.